Live Cookies!

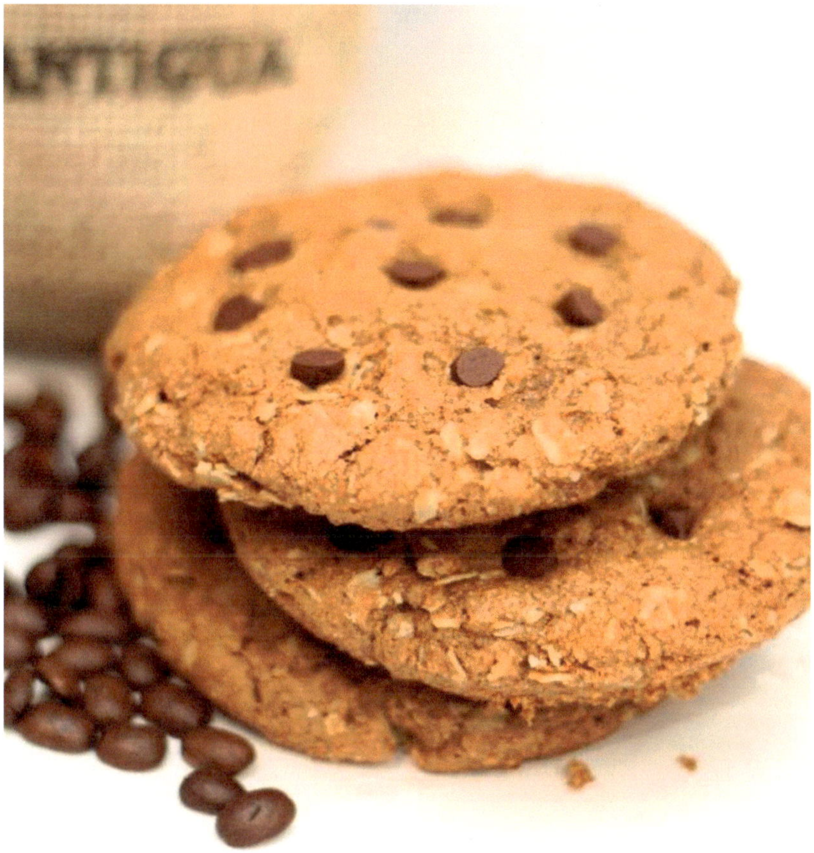

"One Open Aire Market season a gentleman shared with us that his 100 year old mother had begun to eat Live Bread every day and it changed her life for the better.

She was no longer troubled with constipation, and she lived to be 106 years old!"

"Several customers had come to our booth explaining that they were gluten intolerant. We encouraged them to give one of our small loaves a try, just to see. Sure enough, many of our customers that could not eat commercial breads were actually able to enjoy our breads. The fresh grinding and live nutrients had given them bread again."

"One young man was very busy at his job and couldn't get the right foods into his diet. He added a Live Cookie to each day's menu and soon was enjoying better energy and alertness. **Real food feeds bodies**!"

Table of Contents

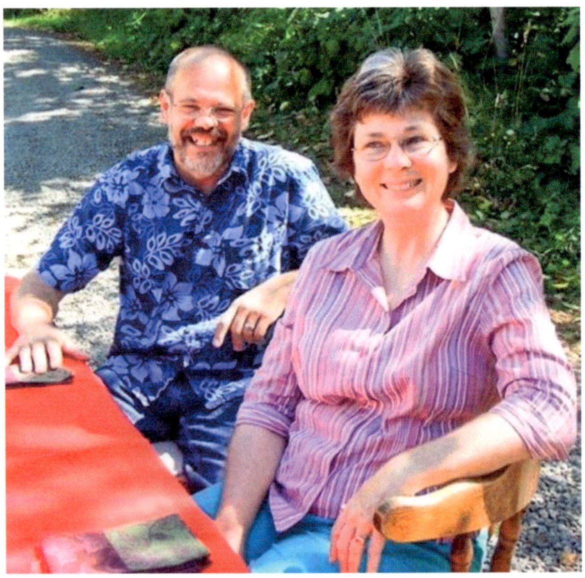

Steve and Sherry Fry

Dear Reader,

Both of us have been faced with life-threatening illnesses and probably would not be alive today were it not for someone who helped us with nutrition.

The recipes in this book, and its basic information were the beginning for us in getting well, and the catalyst that gave us a completely different mindset about food.

Some fundamental areas vital to great health are:

1. *Grains,*
2. *Sweeteners*
3. *Oils*

The general mis-information, about these areas is, frankly, overwhelming!

- What grain is good?
- Why are so many people gluten intolerant?
- Is there a safe sweetener … *anywhere*?
- What is a healthy oil?

As time passed, we got more education and have helped hundreds of other people who thought there was no hope. We wish to share our 17 years of experience with you, and are confident you can apply this knowledge to *your life* in simple ways that will improve your health *forever*.

This book is the first in our "Nutrition From" series to bless our wonderful friends, customers, co-workers, followers, and fans of *The Live Bread Shoppe.*

For 16 wonderful years, the people of Sequim and Western Washington, in the beautiful Pacific Northwest, have blessed us with love and support as we baked and distributed products made with fresh ground flour, extra virgin olive oil, and no refined sweeteners.

We thank you, and we offer this book to you, which, we hasten to add, contains the much sought after secret ***Live Cookie Recipe***!

Read, learn, bake, and live a healthier, happier life!

Steve & Sherry

A Pot of Soup and a Loaf of Bread

This book is intended primarily to teach, debunk myths, and illuminate lives for the purpose of attaining vibrant health. But the fact is, everything's got a beginning story, and this is ours…

About 20 years ago, Steve & Sherry Fry moved to Sequim, Washington. We bought five acres of remote forest, and carved out a home.

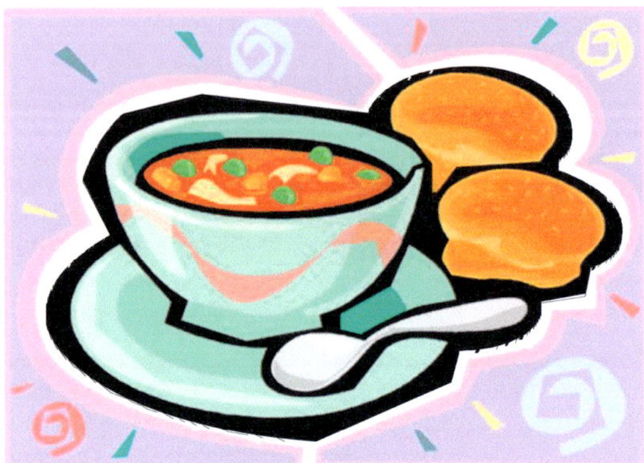

Though there are MANY aspects to this story, right now, we will confine ourselves to those surrounding ***a pot of soup and a loaf of bread.***

Our brand new neighbor, and now long-time friend, Kathie Niclas had just moved into the property above us, along with her wonderful family. Kathie brought us a pot of soup and a loaf of bread.

We frankly don't remember the soup, although we have since had many wonderful bowls from Kathie, but we *do remember* the loaf of bread.

Our family of four – Steve & Sherry, Steven and Julieanne – ate *the whole loaf* in one sitting! That loaf, the beginning of new-found health & The Live Bread Shoppe, was absolutely *delicious*!

Why? Sherry had to know what was different! She had been baking bread for years. using "whole wheat" and "pure vegetable oil," and the like.

Kathie taught her all she knew about freshly ground flour, extra virgin olive oil, and wholesome sweeteners.

The education *did not stop there*! And still hasn't. Kathie started us on a journey that probably won't be over until every member of the Fry Family is pushing up daisies. Steve, Sherry, and both their adult children, along with Esther, their daughter- in-law, are ALL either in, or somehow involved in, living and teaching vibrant health.

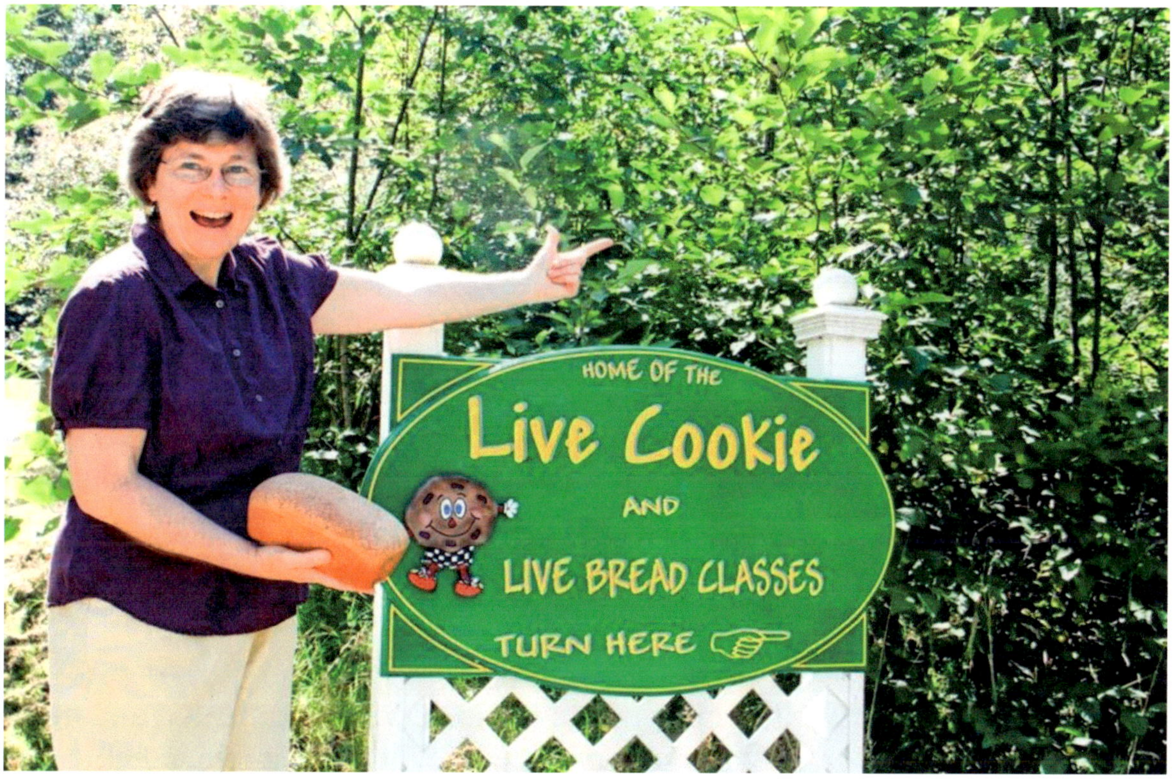

We went on from that pot of soup and a loaf of bread to form the Live Bread Shoppe. We called it "Live" because the vital nutrients were still in the freshness and wholesomeness of the ingredients.

- The flour: Freshly ground.
- The oil: Extra Virgin Olive oil.
- The sweeteners: pure honey or unrefined sugar cane with all the nutrients and minerals still intact.

Although the Live Bread Shoppe closed its doors December 31st, 2012, we continue to serve you with Common Sense Nutritional Therapy: www.CSNtherapy.com

It all started with ***a pot of soup and a loaf of bread.***

Thanks Kathie !

Grain, Gluten, Guts and Good News

Grain

Grain comes in many forms. Some gluten grains are wheat, spelt, oat, and kamut. Some non-gluten grains are teff, amaranth, buckwheat, and quinoa, to name a few.

Let's talk about wheat though, because it's the most well-known and most used.

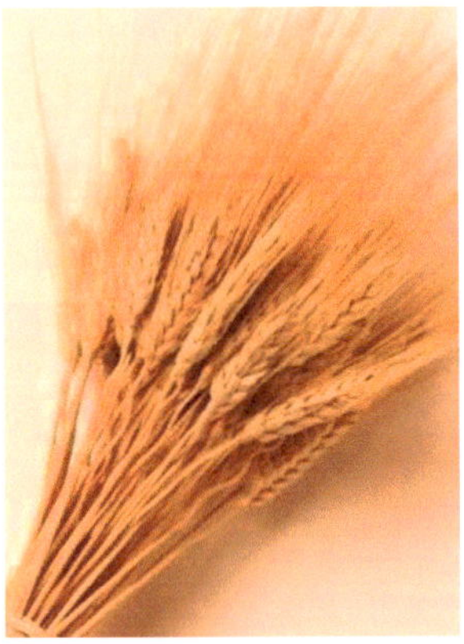

Wheat grows in the field like hay or grass, and its kernels are harvested and stored. The nutrients in wheat can be kept safe for thousands of years, as long as the grain is *not* opened and it is kept *dry*.

Once the grain is opened, there is a 72-hour window before it starts to go bad.

In that time (within 72 hours), protein begins to break down dramatically, and most of the vitamins & minerals are lost through oxidation. Whack an apple in half and you'll see oxidation in a matter of minutes as the apple begins to change colors. The same thing happens with grain, only you don't see it!

Now, ***stop the press***!
Re-read the last paragraph because it can literally change your life.
And it's key to understanding why people have gluten intolerance.

Well over 90% of bread products today are from wheat kernels that were ground months, and even years before they were used to make "fresh" baked goods.

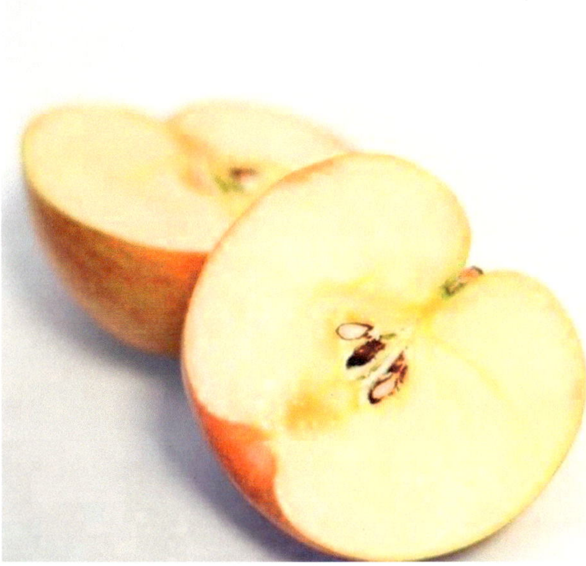

Fresh apple

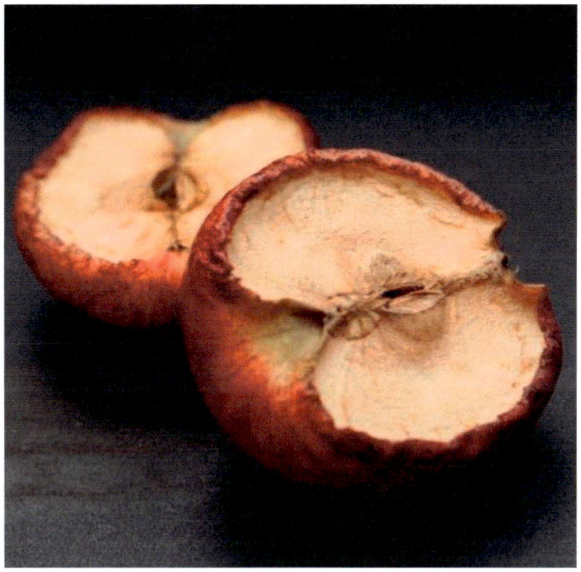

Oxidized apple

Gluten

In the 1900's, the roller mill was invented. It ground wheat and separated the parts. You've heard of them all at some point:

- Wheat gluten,
- Wheat germ, and
- Wheat bran.

The center – the gluten – could now be marketed primarily as white flour. With the germ and the bran gone, it can last for months, even years!

The sad part of the story is that gluten – the center and largest part of the wheat kernel –is only protein. It contains no oil, no vitamins and no minerals.

The roller mill also made white bread possible. White flour is dead. It contains no nutrients and fiber, but it makes for highly marketable flour that can last and last because what would spoil and grow rancid is gone

Guts

In first grade did you get to finger paint? I did, and it was fun!
How about Paper Mache?

Basically, you take plain white flour and water, mix it, and paint it all over stuff you formed out of newspaper. Then it hardens to a tough crust, and you get to color it and take it home to your parents for their admiration.

The interesting thing is the same thing happens in your gut! That's where you absorb all the nutrients from your food.

Your gut has little crevices filled with tiny hairs called cilia. So when you eat some fluffy delicious white bread, it mixes with fluids you ingest, and you get a paper Mache gut.

If it's not too bad, some of the cilia still work, and you're just gluten intolerant.

If it's real bad, you have Celiac disease.
Fancy words for ***you Paper Mache-d your gut.***

So now, you can't eat wheat, you can't absorb your nutrients, and you're probably getting lured into the "gluten free food" maze, which has some of the unhealthiest foods ever created floating around in it, at prices that will break the bank! Well, there is a way out, and it starts with ***real food***, compared to processed "gluten free food!"

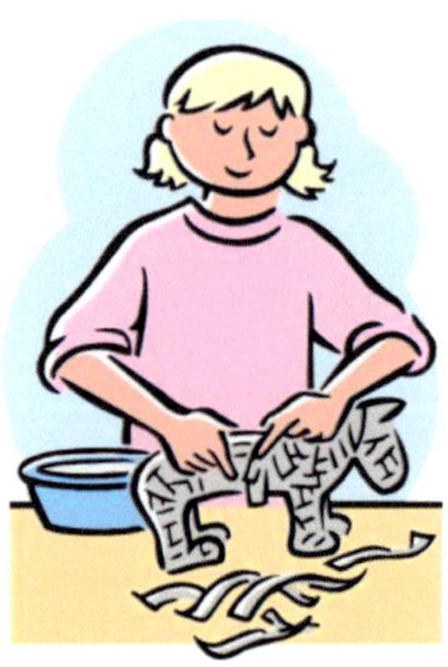

Genetic Modification

Through centuries of hybrid techniques, the gluten content in nearly all wheat grain is unbelievably out of proportion to what God originally intended. Higher gluten content isn't better, it's just more profitable.

If you search online for "GMO," you'll find a lot of information on the effects of genetically modified wheat grain, not something you'd want to eat at all. The subject changes "bad wheat" to "morbid wheat."

Bottom line – get a good organically grown wheat.

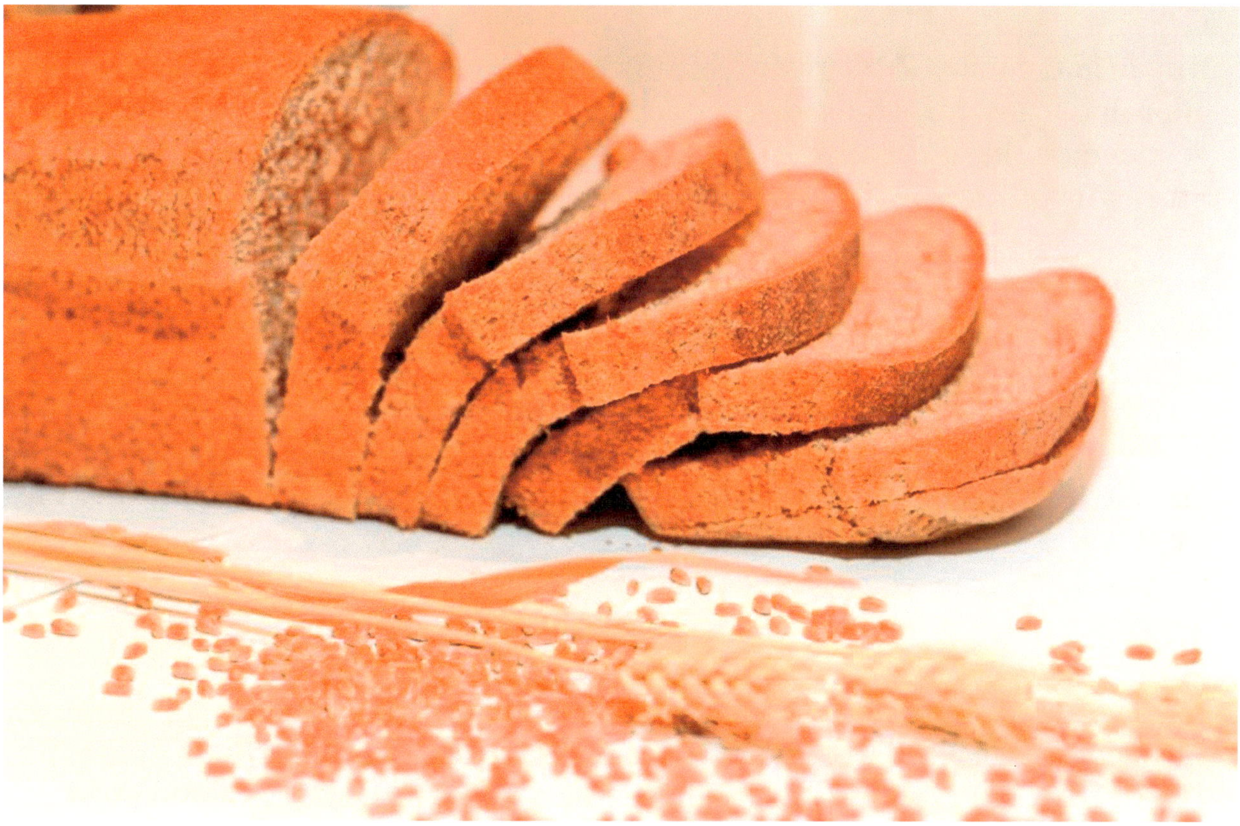

Good News

Now the Good News: Here is some plain, straight, simple advice. If you take it and run with it, you will literally see changes that will astound you! *And it's easier than you might think!*

- **Get a grinder**. This is a valuable investment in your health and the health of your family. Maybe you can split the cost with three other people who live close by.

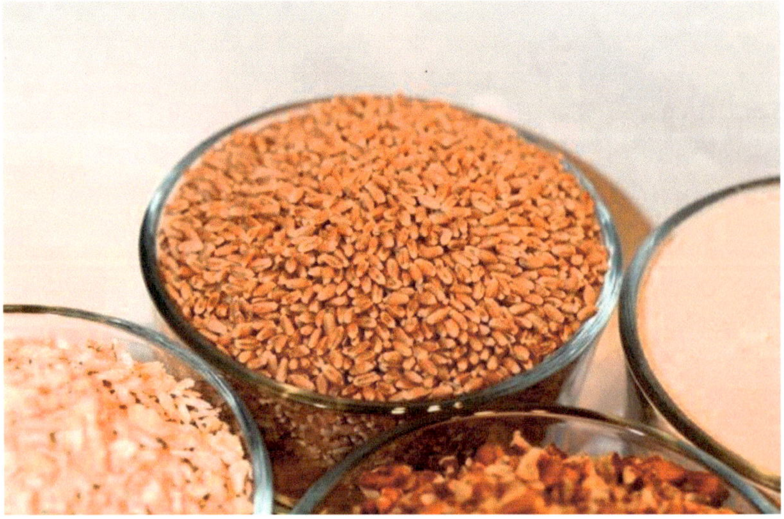

Grind your grain, then freeze it. That stops oxidation.

The refrigerator *will not* stop oxidation. Freezing it will allow many people to buy it and use it together.

(The grinder we have used for two decades is available on our "store" at CSNtherapy.com)

- **Buy organic non-GMO grain**. Spelt is a good alternative to wheat. We eat spelt grain and many non-gluten grains, so if necessary, you don't have to eat wheat to get delicious healthy baked goods.
- **Store all your grain**. You can store grains – not flour – in a dry container until you are ready to grind it. It will keep for a very long time as long as it's dry. If you share grinding with a friend or buy fresh ground flour, then make sure you keep it frozen until use. This will combat oxidation and ensure a healthy gut; and a healthy life!
- **Dairy is good for you** if it's from raw milk. **Beef is good for you** if it's hormone & antibiotic free grass fed beef, and grain is good for you if it's fresh ground and organic. But we Americans need to learn to eat less of these things, ***far less***.
- **Vegetables should be the main** part of every plate. Buy organic, locally grown, if possible, or grow your own alternative permaculture garden. Vegetables should get more attention from you than any other food.
- 80% of your food choices should have ***no ingredients label***.
- **Help your gut heal** by adding *Cultured Foods* into your menu. (In the future, we will dedicate an entire book to cultured foods in our "Nutrition From" series).
- **Drink clean, filtered, non manipulated water**. 48oz per day minimum and make sure you don't "float" your food by drinking too much with a meal. Four ounces should be your maximum water intake during a meal, with all the rest of your daily water intake consumed **away** from food.
- **Remove all *processed*** grains, sweeteners, oils, and salts from your menu.
- **Take steps** to recover your health by reading, taking classes, listening to webinars, and watching videos. We have several suggestions at the end of this book in the "Suggested Reading" chapter.
- Vote with your food dollar by avoiding processed foods and buying whole, unprocessed, fresh and local, healthy food.

Sugar Gone Astray and the Road Back

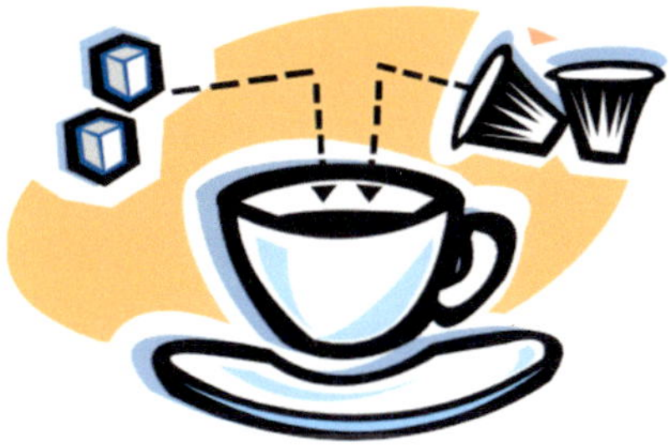

We are convinced that America's number one health problem involves sugar, in all its many forms.

Consider the following:

- Type 2 Diabetes used to be called "Adult Onset Diabetes." Since we now consume more sugar than ever before, it's showing up in toddlers and elementary school children, and it's just referred to as "Type 2 Diabetes."
- High cholesterol is a sugar problem.
- High Fructosc Corn Syrup is harmful.
- One teaspoon of sugar (a soda pop has 12 teaspoons) will reduce your immune function by 50% for up to six hours.
- Synthetic sugar substitutes are, for the most part, among the most deadly substances you could ingest.

The list could go on for pages, but like the title says, there is a "road back." And diabetes can often be reversed or well managed through diet.

Sugar 101

Sugar cane is a stalk that looks a lot like bamboo and grows in very hot climates. There is a product made from sugar cane that is good for you, and then there are **many** that are ***not***.

"Pure cane sugar" is actually dangerous. This is not an exaggeration. The method of manufacturing it involves bleaching, chemicals, and other steps that not only change it from food to "food-like substance," but also poses a serious threat to workers at the sugar plants.

If you become what health professionals call "pre-diabetic," you might be told to supplement your diet with synthesized chromium from the local health food store. But sugar cane, before it's processed, contains the mineral chromium!

Because "pure cane sugar" is in so many products, an average American eats 22 teaspoonfuls of sugar a day!

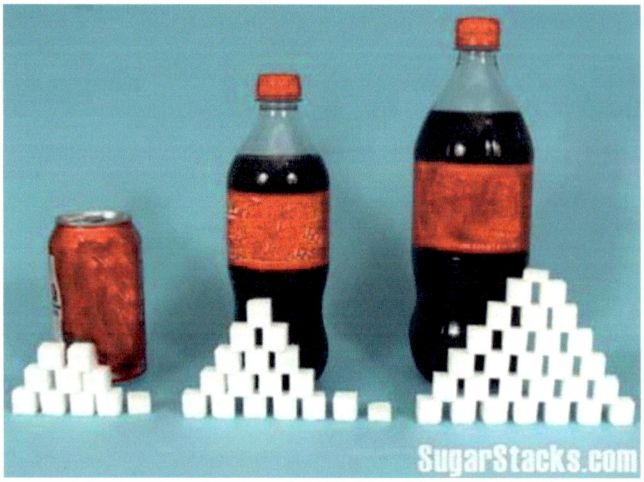

Remember, only one teaspoon of refined white "pure cane sugar" can reduce your immune system by up to 50% for up to six hours! So, what are 22 teaspoons in a day doing to us?

High Fructose Corn Syrup

Other sweeteners such as High Fructose Corn Syrup can have similar harmful effects. If you search online for "the truth about High Fructose Corn Syrup" you will find that the Corn Refiner's Association has many websites touting the benefits of HFCS.

However, Dr. Mark Hyman states that even when HFCS is used in moderation, it is a major cause of:

- Heart disease
- Obesity
- Cancer
- Dementia
- Liver failure

In the words of Dr. Hyman:

HFCS is:

> "…poor-quality, nutritionally depleted, processed industrial food full of empty calories and artificial ingredients."
>
> "If you find "high fructose corn syrup" on the label, you can be sure it is not a whole, real, fresh food full of fiber, vitamins, minerals, phytonutrients and antioxidants.
>
> "Stay away [from HFCS] if you want to stay healthy. We still must reduce our overall consumption of sugar, but with this one simple dietary change you can radically reduce your health risks and improve your health.
>
> "High fructose corn syrup is almost always found in very poor quality foods that are nutritionally vacuous and filled with all sorts of other disease-promoting compounds, fats, salt, chemicals and even mercury."
>
> http://www.huffingtonpost.com/dr-mark-hyman/high-fructose-corn-syrup-dangers_b_861913.html

The Road Back

Sucanat, in its true whole form, is safe, delicious, and healthy. The company "Wholesome Sweeteners" makes it. It is evaporated cane juice. They crush the cane, evaporate the water, and that's it. What's left is a natural product containing all the minerals, including chromium, without the bleaching, chemicals, and other toxins.

Do not get the "blonde" colored Evaporated Cane Juice from Wholesome Sweeteners, because that has had some or all of the molasses removed, which is where the minerals are. Get the ***Sucanat*** only.

Honey, and whole Stevia leaf are other safe sweeteners. Avoid all the chemical sugar alternatives. They are all *very* dangerous to your health and well being. As with grain, be aware that moderate amounts are best.

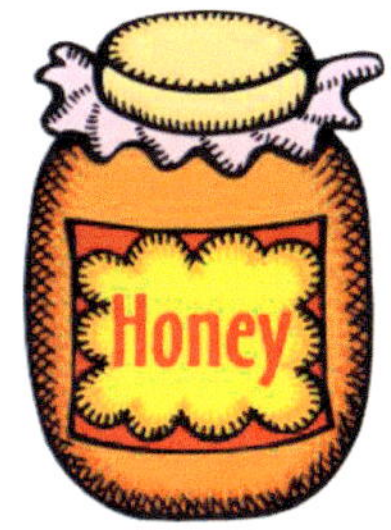

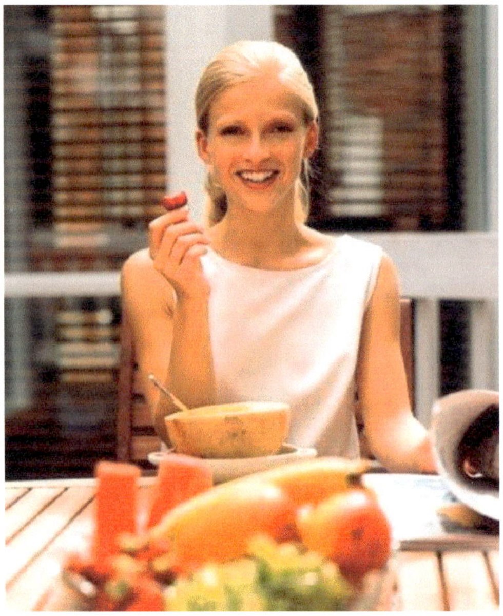

As previously stated, America consumes, per capita, 22 teaspoons per day each.

Even if it's a healthy version, that is outrageously too much! Learn to get the majority of your sweets from fruit: apples, pears, blueberries, blackberries, figs. Other fruits, which have higher natural sugar content, should be consumed sparingly, in small amounts.

Your body will thank you!

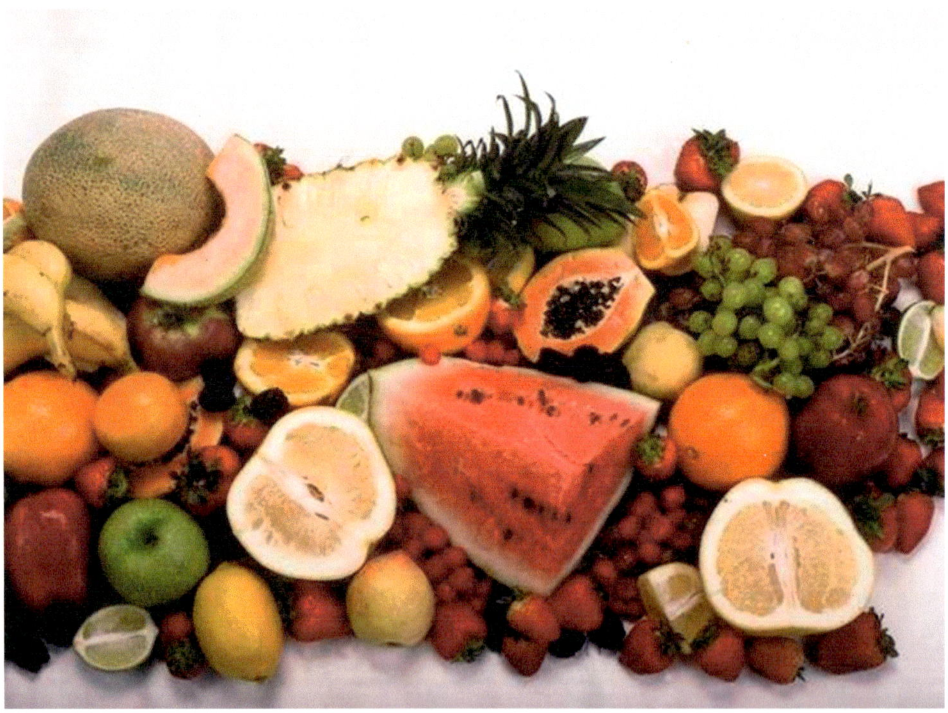

Oil – Slick Lies and an Order of Fries

Good oil is good for you.
Bad oil is bad for you.

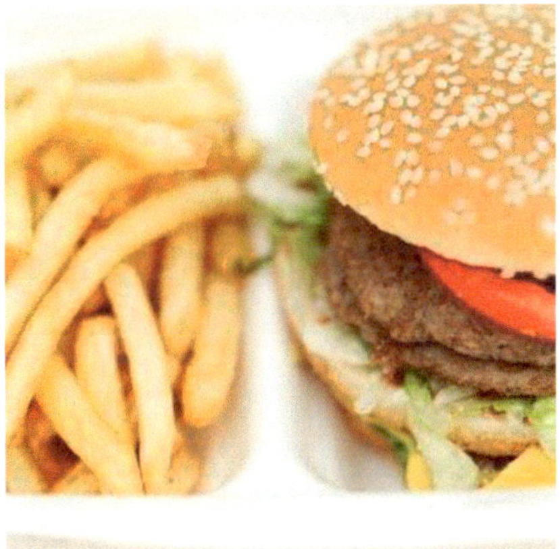

Good oil will give you much needed essential fatty acids for healthy cells.

Bad oil will give you suffocated cells and serious health problems!

The fat-free craze has Americans avoiding all fat, good or bad, including oil.
All oil is *not* created equal.

Since America started the "Fat Free" craze, she has literally become the fattest nation on the planet. People reading labels are putting back *anything* that shows *any* fat! This is a tragedy!

All fat is not created equal, and oil is fat.

Want to Lose Weight?

Then you'd better eat good fat, or your body will get huge while it's looking for the fat it *must* have to survive!

Your brain does not work well without good fat, and that's a fact! Your body will do what it must to get the fat for your brain, your cells, your hormone production, and a whole host of other functions. If you deprive it of those essential fats, the end result is, you will be unhealthy and obese!

So, what do you do? Start eating fries because you heard that you need fat? ***No***! That's the bad fat! The trans fat! The heart attack fat!

Good Fats

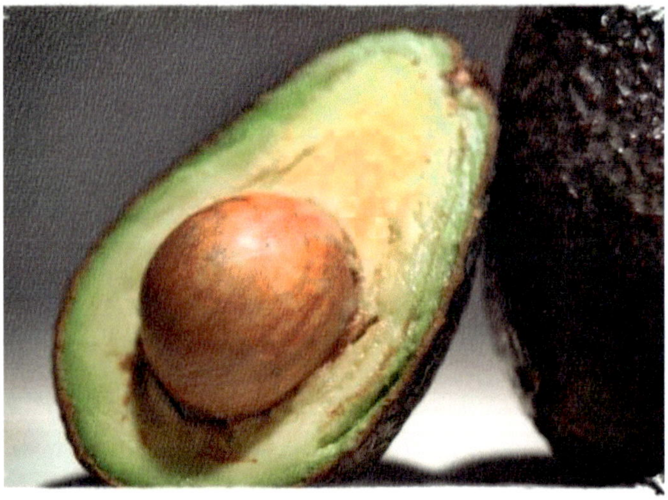

- Extra virgin olive oil
- Unprocessed coconut oil
- Avocados
- Organic butter
- Raw nuts
- Raw seeds

These are all ***good*** fats that you ***must have***.
Eat good fat to gain health and vitality, as well as lose weight.

Bad Fats

- Fried foods
- Almost all vegetable oils
- Margarine
- Hydrogenated oil
- Partially hydrogenated oil

These are some of the *bad* fats that you **must avoid**. Their cumulative use will cause a full scale health crisis, not the least of which will be obesity.

Your body wants to burn fuel, and its favorite fuel is fat … ***good fat***! Fat is also a "life saver" because it serves as a storage case for poisons, excesses, and toxins.

So, the challenge is to clean out the junk, eat the right fats, and then listen to your engine "hum!"

Recipes

So take some of that, and mix it with that other thing, then throw it at the oven, then run….no wait….

Here is Sherry's version: It will be easier than peeling it off the over door. And tastes better too!

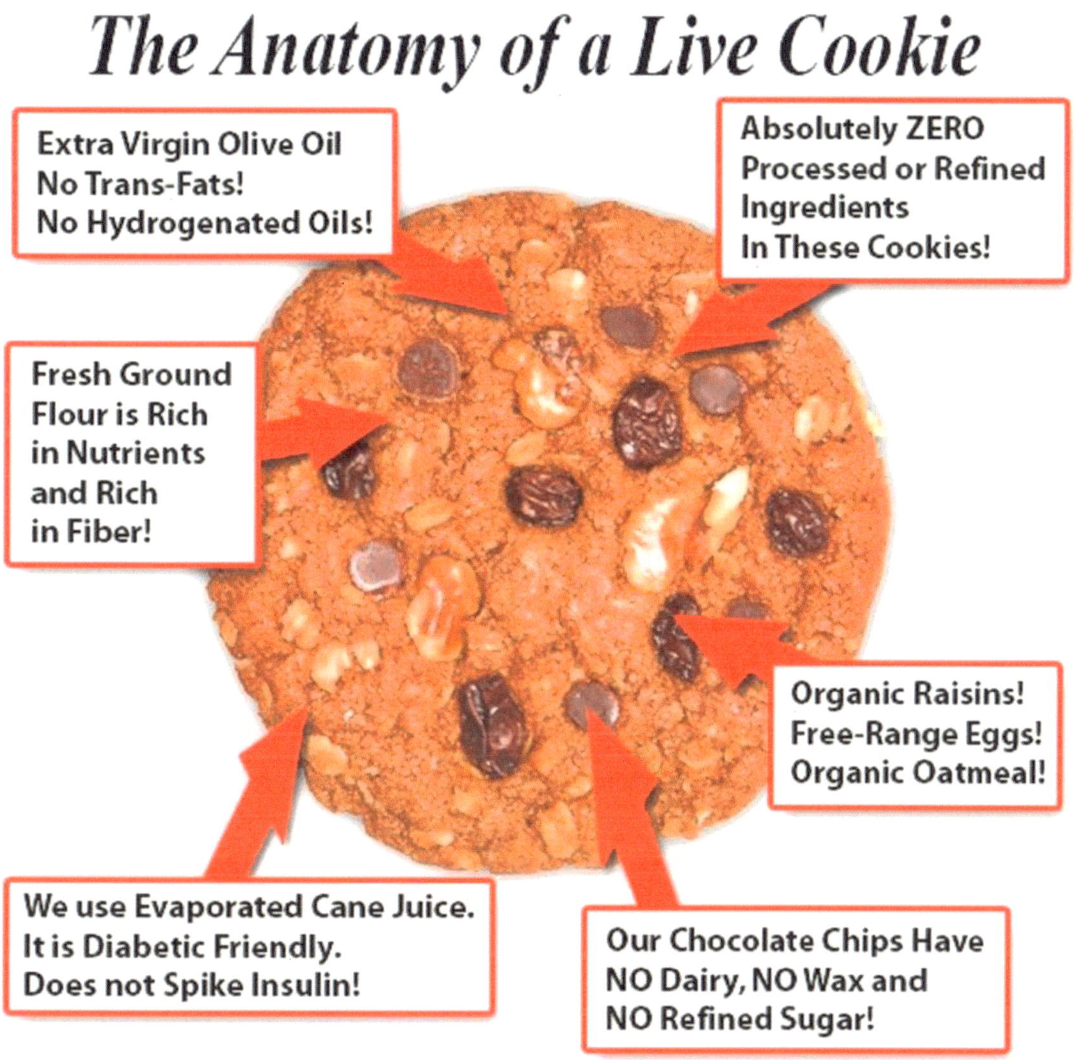

Basic "Live" Cookie Recipe

Makes 24 large or 48 small cookies

Wet: 4 eggs
1 1/2 tsp vanilla

Put the above in a 3 cup measure
Then add extra virgin olive oil to the "2-cup" mark.

Dry: 4 Cups Fresh Ground Red Wheat Flour* (5 cups, if you are using Spelt)
3 Cups Sucanat (**Su**gar **Ca**ne **Nat**ural)
3 Cups Fresh Rolled Oats*
1 1/2 tsp baking soda
1 tsp unprocessed sea salt or Celtic salt

SECRET: I always use a mixer. Put the wet ingredients in the bowl and spin till they are well mixed...till you can't tell them apart any more. Then I thoroughly blend the dry mix and pour it SLOWLY into the wet mix while it's spinning.

I use a wooden spoon to make sure things keep moving. Don't mix too long...only until all the dry ingredients are absorbed and become like cold ice cream in consistency. Then stop, do NOT over mix. You can use a hand mixer, but the job is more difficult. Make sure the wet is well mixed before adding the dry. Add the dry ingredients slowly...this is a MUST.

Use an ice cream scoop (medium to small size) and make balls with the dough. Once on the pan, flatten gently to make a small patty-like shape. If you do not use the pre-formed cookie pans, then leave plenty of room between so they can spread without touching.

Bake at 325° for 19-21 minutes in a conventional oven, or 15-17 minutes in a convection oven. They are done when there is substance to the touch, but the whole cookie is still somewhat soft.

The rest of the cooking happens in the pan, outside the oven while they cool. Be careful not to overcook.

Voila! You have now made a Live Cookie!

**Both wheat and oats should be fresh milled.*

Grind wheat in a home mill: "Wonder Mill."
Buying flour or oatmeal in the store means you are not getting food.
Invest in your health and get the tools you need to do it right.
Oat groats and wheat kernels keep indefinitely when unopened and kept dry.

Roll oats in an Oak Flaker or Roller.
The mill is available on our website. www.CSNtherapy.com/store/store-main.html
The flaker is available online. http://oatflaker.com

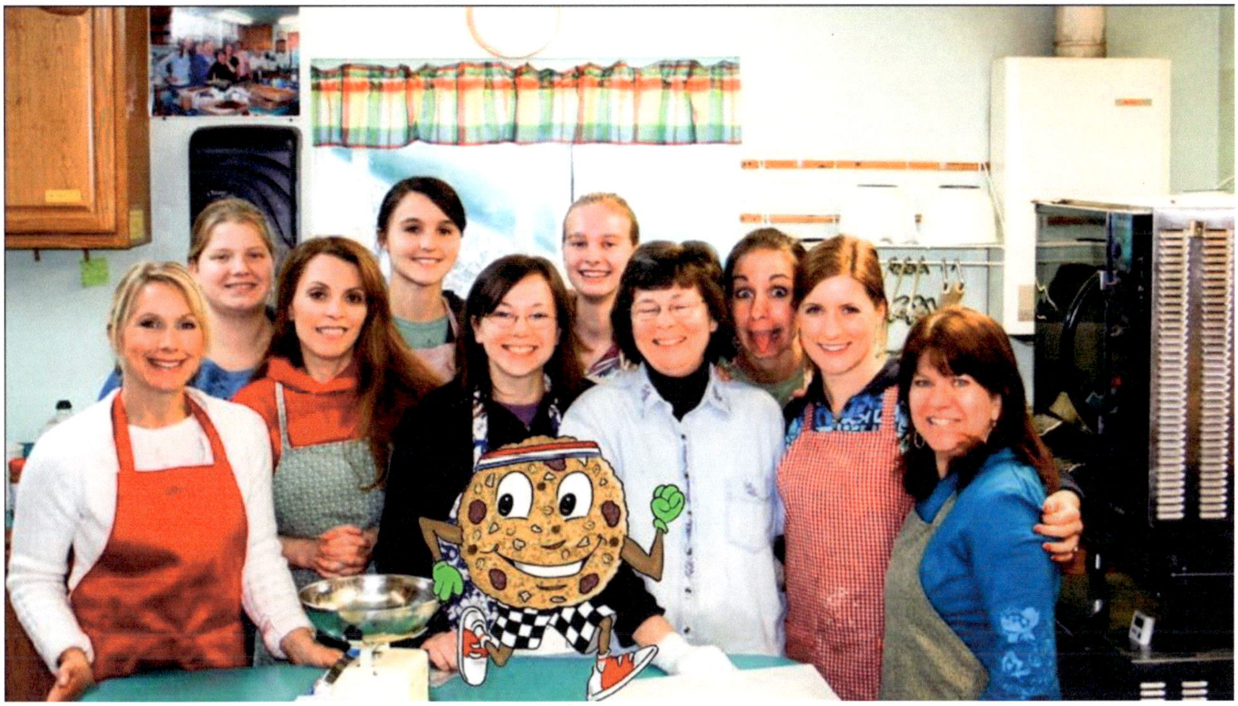

Gluten-Free Recipes

To make your recipes gluten-free, combine buckwheat, amaranth and teff. Be sure to combine all three flours before measuring for a recipe.

2 cups Buckwheat
2 cups Amaranth
1 cup Teff

(This makes 5 cups of flour)

Cookie Variations

You can add up to one cup of ingredients (combined) to the basic cookie recipe without changing ratios.

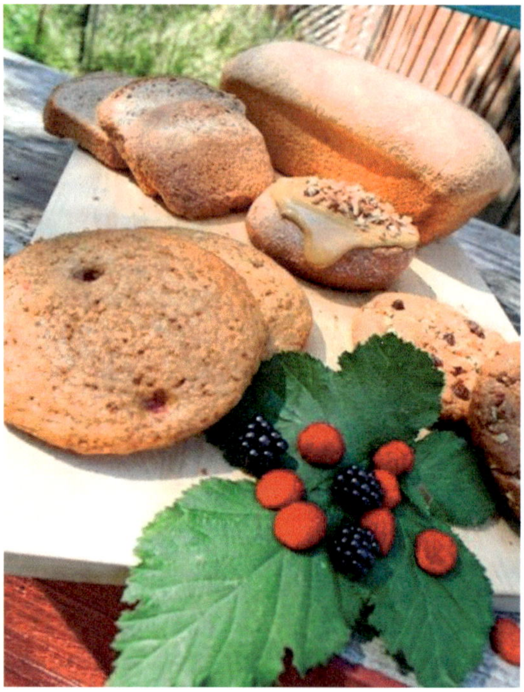

Apple Cranberry

To the Basic Recipe add:

1/2 cup dried apple pieces, 1/2 cup dried cranberries (always use the ones sweetened with apple juice, not sugar) – spin the dried fruit in the wet mixture before adding the dry to help separate the pieces well.

Add 1/2 tsp nutmeg, 1/8 tsp mace and 2 tsp cinnamon to the dry mix. Continue with rest of directions for the Basic recipe.

Ginger

To the Basic Recipe add: 5 tsp ginger root powder, 1 1/2 tsp allspice, 1 1/2 tsp cloves and 1 tsp cinnamon to the dry mix, stir in well, then follow the Basic Recipe from here.

Lemon Pecan and **Orange Chocolate Chip**

Very simple—add 1 tbsp of either lemon or orange. Add either 2/3 cup pecan pieces or 2/3 chocolate chips. If it is a wet ingredient, add to wet, if dry, add to dry and then just follow the Basic recipe from there. Easy!

The Original

To the dry part of the Basic Recipe, simply add equal amounts of healthy chocolate chips, walnut pieces and raisins– equal to a combined total of one cup (or you can put these items in by hand on top after making the basic recipe). Leave these items out all together and simple make the Basic Recipe and you have **Vanilla Oatmeal**.

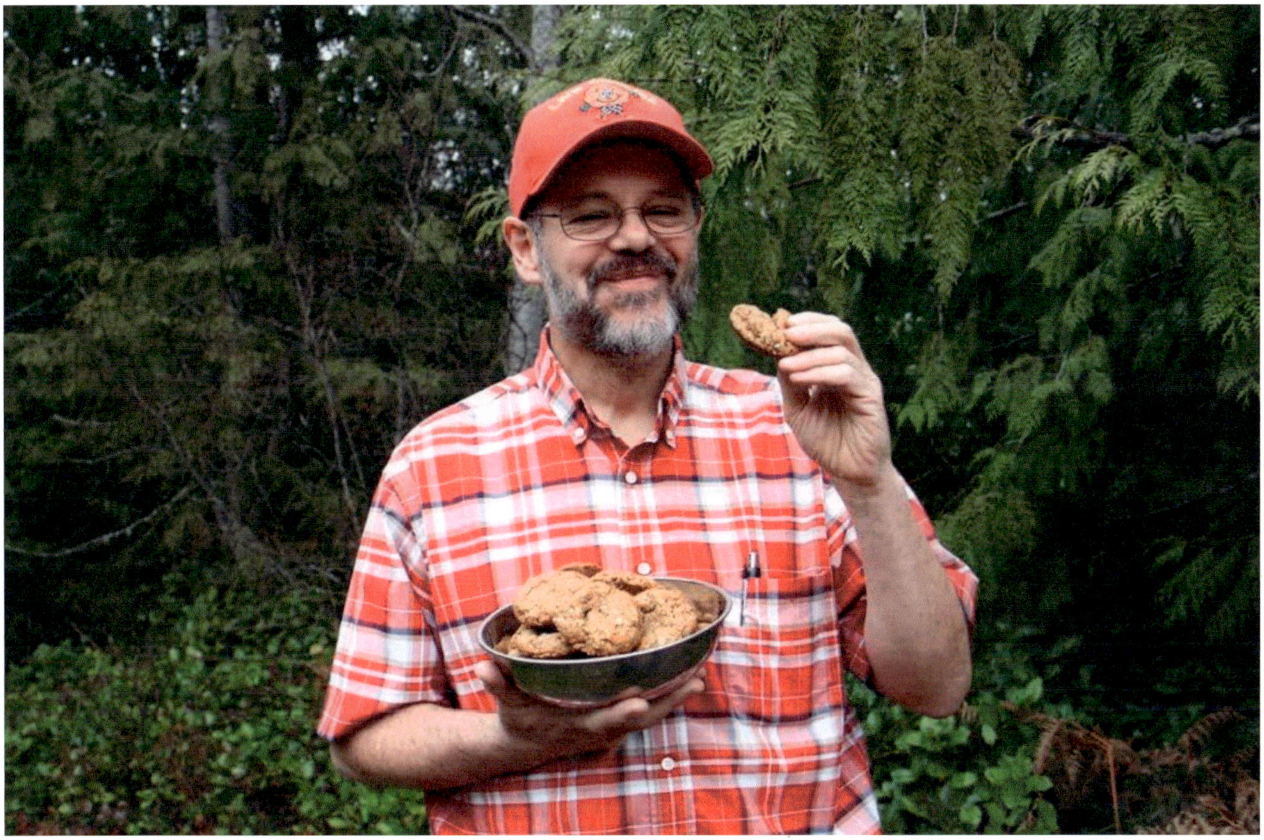

Pumpkin Spice

Add 1/4 cup pumpkin puree to the wet part of the Basic Recipe and spin till well mixed in. Add 2 tsp cinnamon, 2 tsp ginger, 2 tsp nutmeg, and 1 tsp allspice to the dry mix and stir in well before adding to wet. Mix carefully, will be a bit sticky. Bake and enjoy.

Peanut Butter Swirl

This one is a bit tricky. Make these changes to the Basic Recipe:

Use two cups oats instead of three. Add 3/4 cup quality cocoa powder. Begin the basic recipe. As the dough is finishing, dollop in 3/4 cup freshly ground peanut butter. Make sure you watch closely and only let it partially mix in. These cookies will be delicate and the peanut butter should be in globs through the mix. Place in pans, add chocolate chips on top and bake as usual.

Peanut Butter Chocolate Chip*

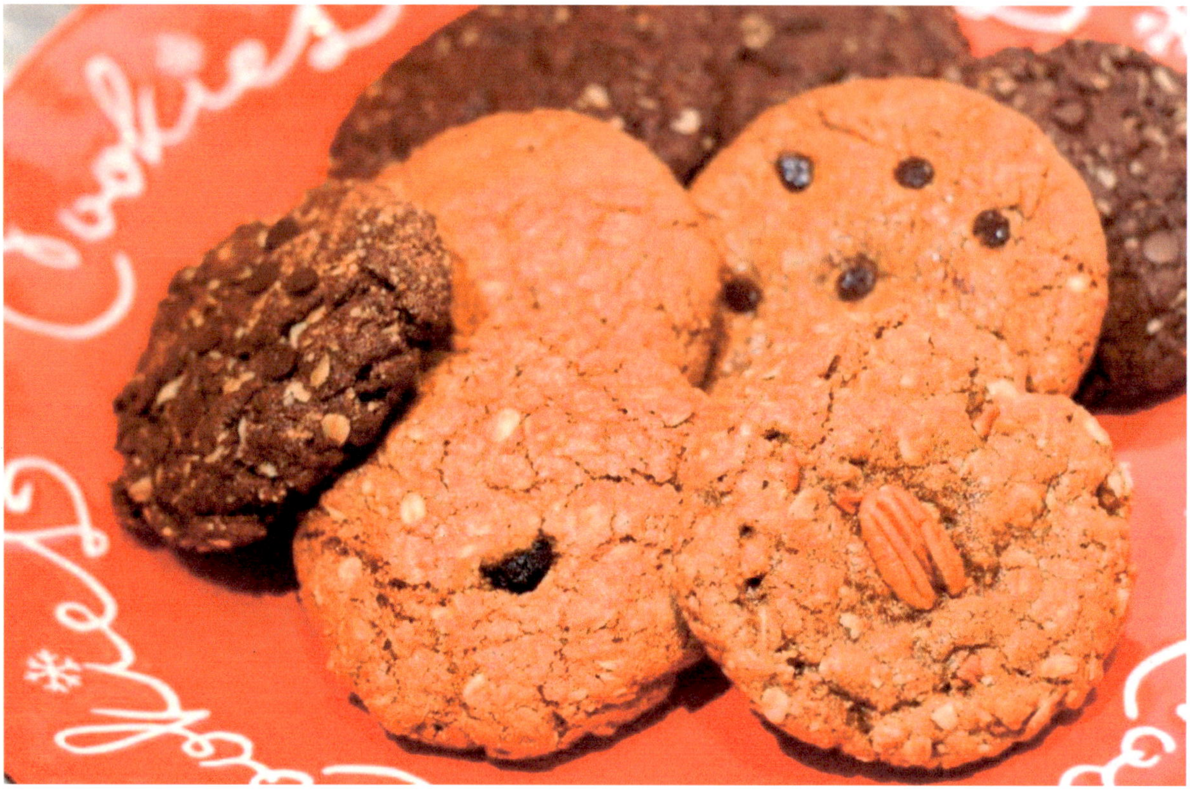

Leave the oats out completely, reduce the oil to 1 3/4, and mix one cup peanut butter into the wet mix until well blended. Add dry ***very*** slowly and mix carefully, it gets ready quickly. Put in pans, add chocolate chips.

*May substitute Almond Butter for this variation.
Adding 2 tsp of almond flavoring is also nice.

Peppermint Cocoa Chocolate Chip

Leave the peanut butter out, keep the oats at 3 cups, and the cocoa at 3/4 cup and add 1 to 2 teaspoons peppermint oil flavoring and chocolate chips, in or on top.

Have fun finding some of your own variations and eat the cookies that bring health in every bite!

Buckwheat Chocolate Chip Cookie

It's wheat free, gluten free, diary free and can be egg-free:

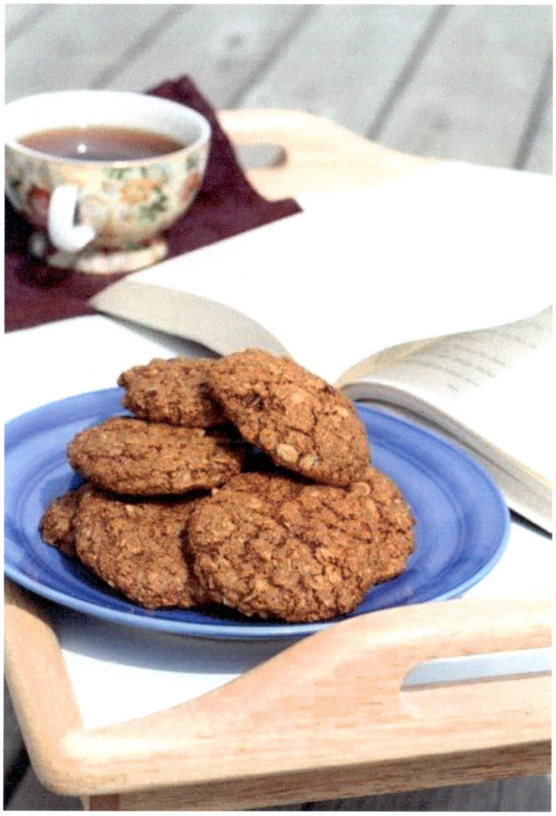

Wet: 4 eggs*
1 1/2 tsp vanilla
Up to 2 cup line with Extra Virgin Olive Oil

Dry: 3 cups Sucanat
2 cups Buckwheat (fresh ground) 2
cups Amaranth (fresh ground)
1 cup Teff (fresh ground—pour slowly in grinder)
1/4 C flaxseed (fresh ground—coffee mill works)
¼ C almonds (ground to small pieces)
1 3/4 cup small coconut flakes
1 1/2 tsp baking soda
1 tsp unprocessed sea salt or Celtic salt

Now follow same directions as the Basic Recipe.

**If you would like to make it eggless, then remove the ground flaxseed from the dry ingredients, increase the coconut flakes by 1/4 cup, then use the following Flaxseed Egg Replacement in place of the 4 eggs:*

Flaxseed Egg Replacement
4 eggs=1/2 cup ground flaxseed, and it will be very gelatin-like.
1 cup hot water. Blend and let stand 15 minutes, then use in place of the eggs.

(To replace only one egg, use 2 tbsp ground flaxseed and 1/4 cup hot water)

Some Buckwheat Cookie Variations

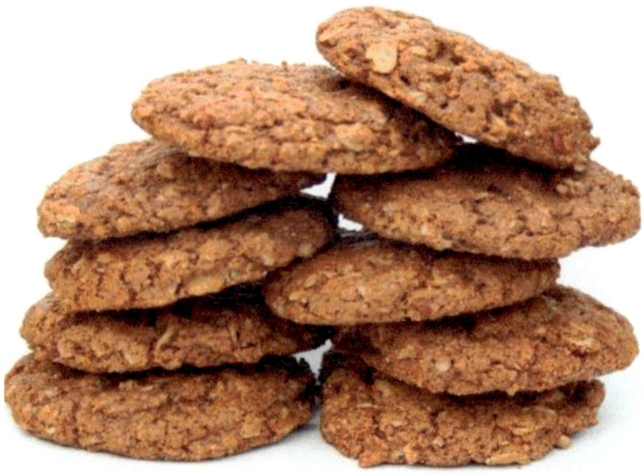

Lemon Pecan

Trade out the chocolate chips and almonds for 1 TBSP lemon flavoring and 1/4 cup pecans pieces.

Then follow the basic recipe directions.

Ginger

Keep the almonds in, take out the chocolate chips and put in these spices:

5 tsp ground ginger, 1/12 tsp cloves, 1 1/2 tsp allspice, 1 tsp cinnamon, then follow the basic recipe directions.

Chocolate Walnut

Replace 1 cup of amaranth with 3/4 cup of quality unsweetened cocoa powder. Replace the almonds pieces with walnut pieces: 2/3 cup walnuts.

Then follow the basic recipe directions.

Almond Chocolate Chip

Replace oatmeal with 3 cups coconut, small flakes. Add 1 to 2 tsp almond flavoring. Add ¾ cup diced almonds. Keep 2/3 cup chocolate chips.

Marathon Cookie

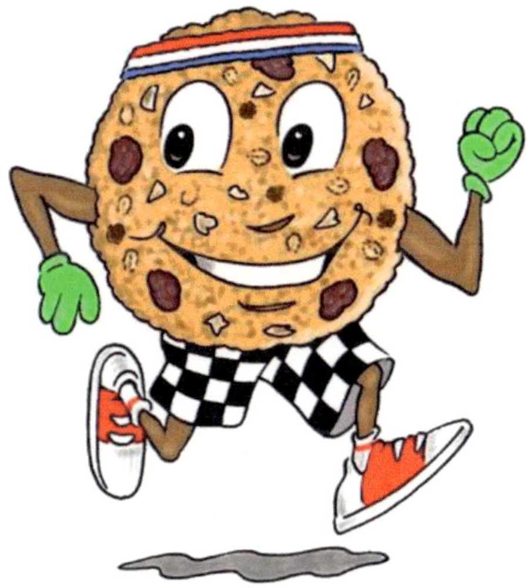

- 2 cups fresh rolled oats
- 3/4 cup pecan pieces (small)
- 2/3 cup sunflower seeds (raw)
- 1/4 cup almond pieces (small)
- 1/8 cup sesame seeds

- 1/3 cup apricot pieces (small)
- 1/3 cup raisins
- 1/3 cup dates (rolled in oat flour)

- 1/8 tsp mace
- 2 level tablespoons ground coriander

Combine fresh rolled oats (roll them yourself; everything in the store is oxidized) almond chunks, pecan pieces, walnut pieces, sunflower seeds, sesame seeds in a bowl; use in place of the oatmeal in basic recipe.

Then combine the dried fruit in a bowl; add all to dry ingredients, blend in spices, then mix as stated in the Basic Recipe.

Option: put healthy chocolate chips on top, then bake!

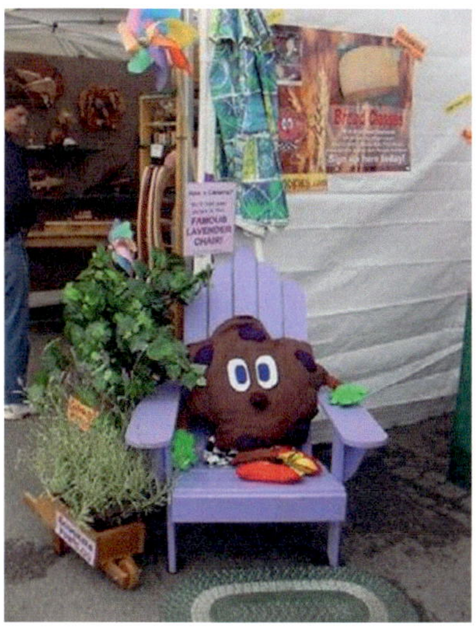

Our Marathon Live Cookie Guy puppet was a great eye catcher at the Sequim Lavender Festival for several years in a row. We actually did make Lavender cookies and found that Lavender, Lemon and Cranberry made a great combo.

(In 2007 we were the official cookie for the North Olympic Discovery Marathon)

Whole Wheat Bread Recipe (Makes four loaves)

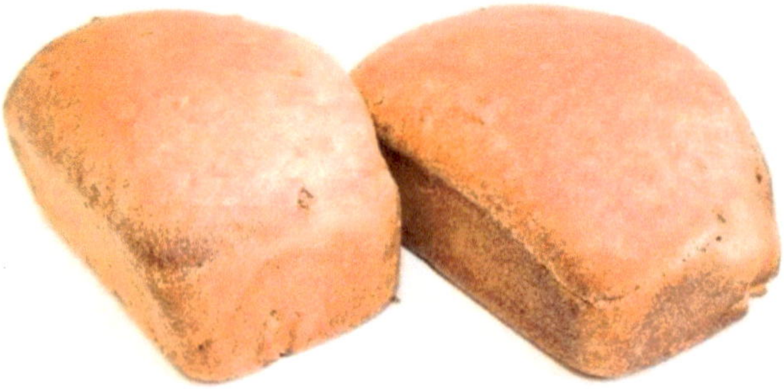

Grind 9 Cups Of Wheat Berries (Equal To 13 Cups Of Flour)

If flour is frozen, bring to room temperature first

Wet Ingredients: 5 cups very warm water (not higher than 105°)

- 1/2 cup extra virgin olive oil
- 1/3 cup honey
- 3 tsp sea salt
- 2/3TBSP active dry yeast (I have used SAF yeast for years, works great!)

Put wet ingredients in mixer bowl:

- Turn on mixer—low speed
- Add ½ of the ground flour (6 1/2 Cups)
- Add yeast; do not put yeast directly into water for this application.

(If you are proofing the yeast first, then make sure temperature is less than 105° but not below 98°)

- Blend at high speed for 1 minute.

(If flavorings such as raisins, nuts, spices desired, this is the place to add them)

Add rest of flour, mix on low speed:

- Set timer to mix for 7 minutes, on low speed.
- Allow dough to rest for 2 – 5 minutes in mixer.
- Punch down by a quick stir in mixer.
- Roll Out On Oiled Board
- Shape into 4 loaves (use oil to handle; do not use more flour; do not knead)

Place in pans and let rise till double; bake at 350°

30-35 minutes in conventional gas oven. 33 minutes in convection gas oven (if using electric ovens, shorten the time by 5 minutes). Bottom should thump, sides should feel firm to a gentle squeeze when done.

NOTE: A Bosch or Kitchen aid can be used, but it must be halved -- the recipe for half follows:

Whole Wheat Bread Recipe (Makes two loaves)

(For any variations, cut added ingredients in half)

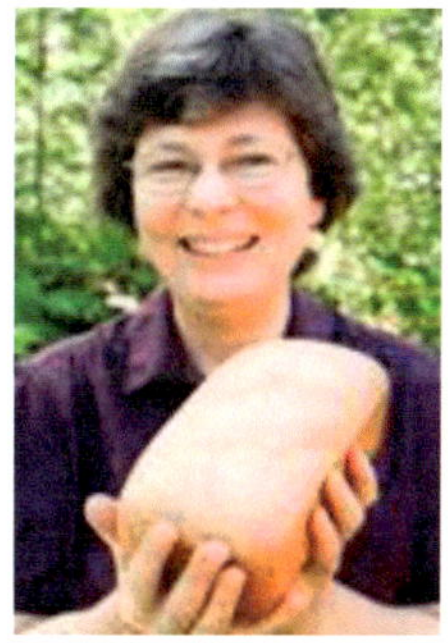

For use with a Kitchen Aide or smaller mixer:

Grind 4 1/2 cups of wheat berries
(Equal to 6 ½ - 6 2/3 cups of flour)
(if flour is frozen, bring to room temperature first)

2 ½ cups very warm water (105° to 110°)
1/4 cup olive oil
1/4 cup honey
1 ½ tsp sea salt
(Put above ingredients into mixcr and spin)
Add ½ the flour amount and 2 TBSP active dry yeast

Spin mixer again, till yeast is well distributed in the liquid dough
Add rest of flour and set timer for 6 minutes on LOWEST setting
(Kitchen-Aides tend to be more aggressive, so we lower the time to help the dough form without over-mixing.)

Once mixture is well kneaded, remove from bowl, pour out onto an oiled board or counter. Shape into loaves. Handle just enough to shape them (but no more) so gluten is not over-worked.

Let rise to double.

Bake in oven at 350° for 25-35 minutes for regular sized loaves.
Bake 20-30 minutes for smaller loaves.
Electric ovens may need a bit more time.
Convection ovens may need a bit less.

Rosemary Thyme Bread

Follow the "BASIC' bread recipe and add the following:

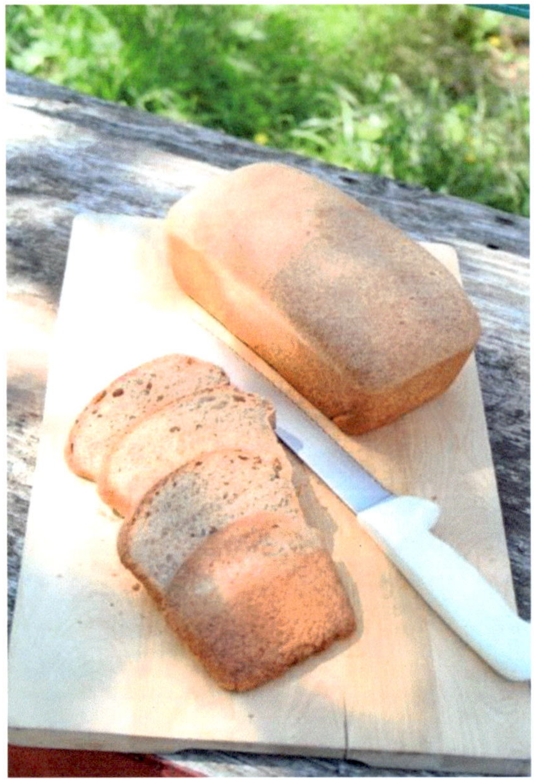

2/3 cup grated carrot
(pressed dry in a paper towel)

2/3 cup grated zucchini
(pressed dry in a paper towel)

1 tsp ground rosemary

1 1/2 tsp thyme leaf

1 1/2 tsp rosemary leaf

Apple Pecan Cranberry Bread

Follow the "BASIC" bread recipe and add these following ingredients:

2/3 cup pecans pieces, chopped small

2/3 cup dried apples—packed tight

2/3 cup dried cranberries—packed tight
(watch sugar on this; get the ones sweetened with apple juice)

2/3 raisins—packed tight

Cinnamon Roll Variation

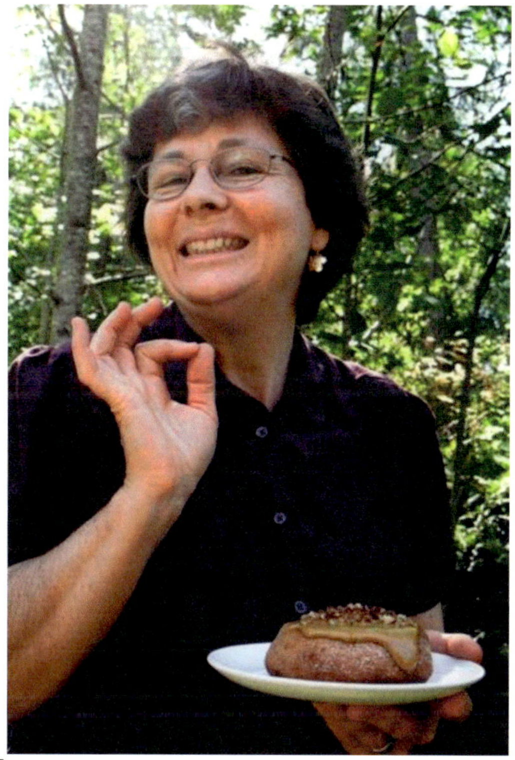

1 cup Sucanat
2 – 3 tsp cinnamon
1 stick of organic butter, melted 2/3—
3/4 cup raisins

Make the Basic Recipe and roll out the dough on a cutting board. Melt organic butter, spread over entire dough, then add cinnamon, Sucanat and raisins.

Roll up, cut with thread, place sideways in baking pan, close together. Bake 20+ minutes at 350. When center springs back they are done. Frost with cream cheese frosting.

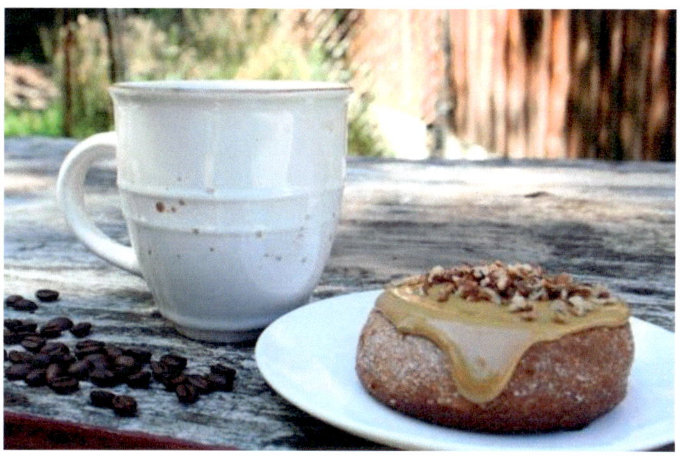

Cream Cheese Frosting

Half pint Nancy's cream cheese
3/4 cup Sucanat
Blend in a bowl with hand mixer till creamy and smooth.

Apply to tops of rolls.

Try to get everything organic when possible.

Muffin Recipe

(Makes 12 large muffins or 24 small muffins, or 2 loaves of Quick Bread)

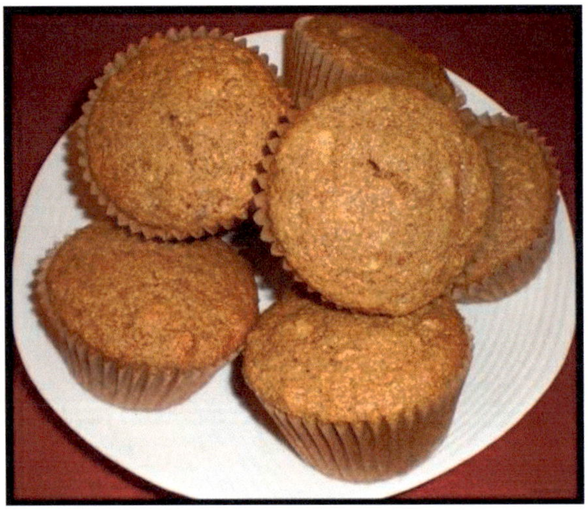

3 cups fresh ground flour*
1 cup sucanat
1 tsp sea salt
4 tsp baking powder

3 eggs
1 1/3 cups water
2/3 cup extra virgin olive oil

Assemble wet ingredients in a bowl, mix with a wire whip, and set aside.

Mix dry ingredients in a separate bowl. Add flavorings such as raisins, nuts, chocolate chips, frozen fruit to dry ingredients, mix in gently so everything is coated with flour. Do not add more than 1 cup, combined, of desired dry flavorings.

Add liquid flavorings (such as orange, lemon or peppermint flavorings, mashed banana) up to 4 tsp to taste, in wet bowl before blending.

Stir the dry into the wet gently just until everything is wet. Do not over-mix or muffins will be tough and flat.

Pour batter into muffin pans. Bake at 400° for 13-16 minutes.
Muffins are done when they spring back to the touch. This recipe works really well using Muffin Topper pans. Cooks faster, much fluffier.

*Notes on flour:

- If using wheat, use 3 cups of flour.
- If using spelt or kamut use 3 3/4 cups of flour.
- To make gluten-free, simply use the Gluten-Free flour combo on page 19 in place of the wheat flour.

For Quick Bread: Pour batter into two loaf pans. Bake at 375 degrees for 35-45 minutes (depending on oven), or until the top springs back.

Suggested Reading

Nourishing Traditions
by Sally Fallon

Health Hazards of White Sugar
by Lynne Melcombe

The Sugar Trap and How to Avoid it
by Beatrice Trum Hunter (out of print)

Fats that Heal, Fats that Kill
by Udo Erasmus

Choosing the Right Fats
by Udo Erasmus

Adrenal Fatigue, the 21st Century Stress Syndrome
by James L. Wilson, ND, DC, PhD

Know Your Fats: *The Complete Primer for Understanding the Nutrition of Fats, Oils, & Cholesterol,*
By Mary G. Enig, PhD

A Whole Foods *Primer*
by Beatrice Trum Hunter

About the Authors

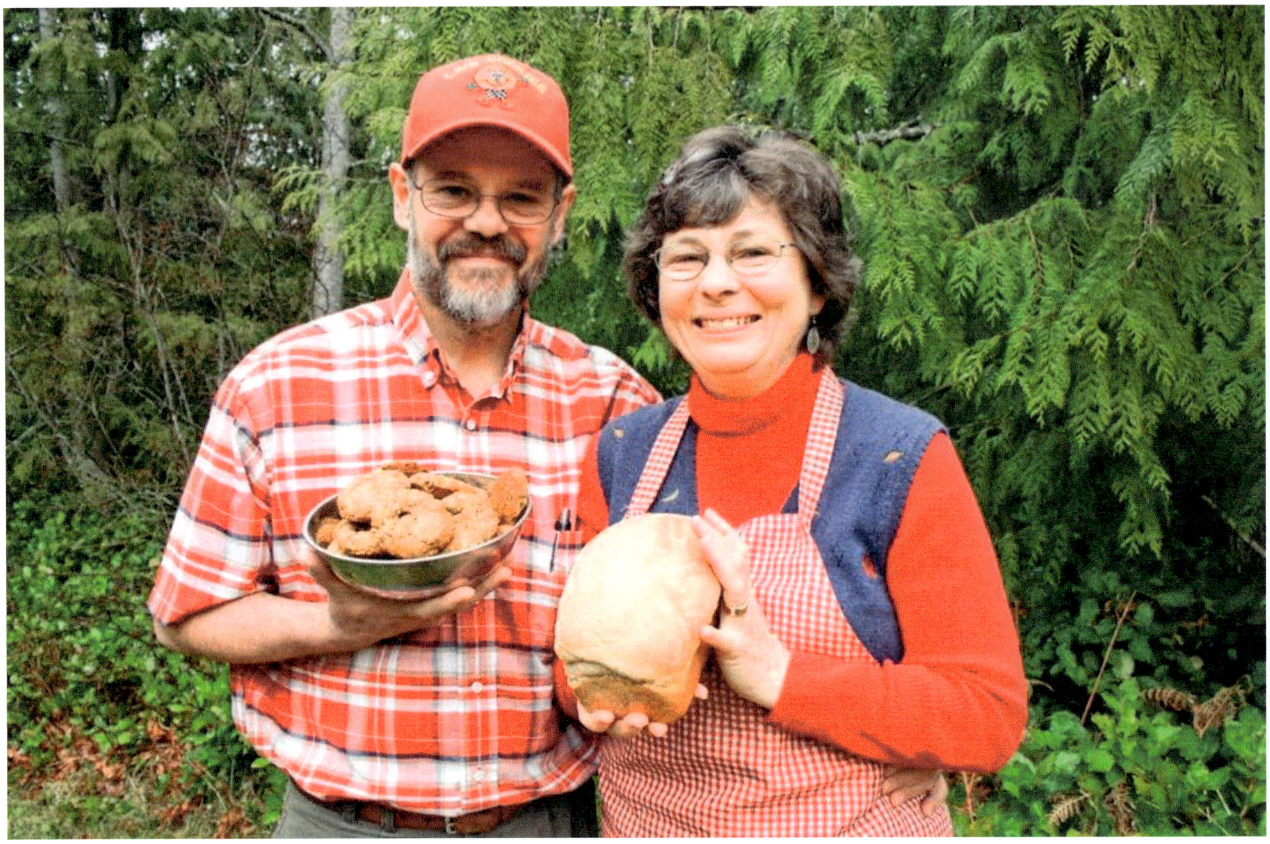

Steve & Sherry Fry own and operate "Common Sense Nutritional Therapy".

Steve and Sherry are BOTH Certified Healing Food Specialists. Additionally, Sherry is a Functional Nutritional Therapy Practitioner

Details about services and classes are available at CSNtherapy.com

Steve & Sherry have two grown children. Steven is married to Esther, and they live with their 2 children in Florida. Julieanne married to Ramoth Gilead and travel the United States sharing their original music.

Steve and Sherry constantly add to their nutritional education and continue to share their discoveries in classes, and through DVD's. Their first DVD, the "Bread Class DVD," is available at www.CSNtherapy.com, in the "store."

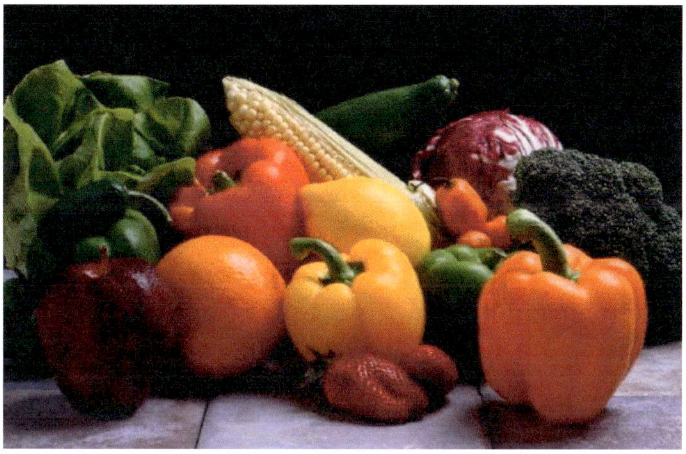

Health is a valuable privilege and learning to take proper care of it has become the core of their passion.

As a family they want to enjoy vibrant health and help others do the same.

The Fry's are on a journey. Their chapter in Sequim has now come to a close. They are stepping into the next chapter and seeking to help many more in their new clinic and classroom in Puyallup, Washington.

To contact the Fry's, please visit their website at **www.CSNtherapy.com**:

- DVDs – a full "Live Bread" instructional workshop is available
- Classes
- Workshops
- Health consultations
- Permaculture gardens

Edited by Allan Harris and Sally M. Harris
Cover design by Sally M. Harris
Photos courtesy of Julianne Marie, Sonlit Photography

Made in the USA
Monee, IL
12 September 2026

62979092R00021